THE COMPLETE KIDNEY TRANSPLANT DIET COOKBOOK

A Flavorful Guide to Nourishing Your Well-Being Post Transplant, to Manage and Improve Renal Functions and to Prevent Complications

By

Dr. Donna Matias

Table of Contents

Introduction

Welcome Message

Welcome to "The Complete Kidney Transplant Diet Cookbook" – a culinary guide designed to inspire and support you on your journey to a vibrant and healthy life post-kidney transplant.

Embarking on a new chapter after a kidney transplant can be both exciting and challenging. We understand the importance of adopting a nourishing and enjoyable diet that complements this significant phase of your health journey. This cookbook is crafted with care, offering a diverse array of recipes meticulously curated to align with the specific dietary considerations that come with post-transplant life.

In these pages, you'll discover more than just recipes – you'll find a companion on your path to wellness. From wholesome breakfasts to delightful desserts, each recipe is thoughtfully created to cater to your nutritional needs while tantalizing your taste buds. The ingredients are carefully chosen to align with the guidelines that support kidney health, ensuring a harmonious balance between flavor and well-being.

Remember, this cookbook is not just about what's on your plate; it's about embracing a lifestyle that celebrates health, vitality, and the joy of savoring delicious, kidney-friendly meals. As you explore these recipes, we encourage you to personalize them to suit your preferences and dietary requirements. Moreover, always consult with your healthcare professionals for personalized advice on your unique health journey.

We hope this cookbook becomes an integral part of your kitchen, fostering a love for cooking and eating that promotes not only physical wellness but also a sense of satisfaction and joy. Welcome to a world of flavorful and kidney-conscious delights – let the cooking adventure begin!

Understanding the Importance of Diet After Kidney Transplantation

Kidney transplantation marks a transformative milestone in the lives of individuals with kidney disease. While the surgery itself is a crucial step towards improved health, the journey doesn't end there.

Post-transplantation, adopting a mindful and tailored diet becomes an integral aspect of maintaining kidney health and ensuring the success of the transplant.

The Role of Nutrition:

Supporting Healing and Recovery:

Adequate nutrition plays a vital role in the healing process post-surgery. Nutrient-rich foods contribute to tissue repair and overall recovery.

Minimizing Medication Side Effects:

Immunosuppressive medications, crucial for preventing organ rejection, may have side effects such as weight gain, bone loss, and changes in blood sugar levels. A well-balanced diet can help manage these effects.

Maintaining Optimal Organ Function:

A kidney-friendly diet assists in maintaining optimal function of the transplanted kidney by controlling factors like blood pressure and fluid balance.

Dietary Considerations:

Sodium and Fluid Control:

Managing sodium intake helps regulate blood pressure and fluid balance, reducing the risk of swelling and high blood pressure.

Protein Intake:

Adequate but not excessive protein intake is essential for healing, muscle maintenance, and overall body function. A balance needs to be struck to avoid placing undue stress on the kidneys.

Phosphorus and Potassium Regulation:

Controlling phosphorus and potassium intake is crucial as imbalances can lead to complications. Transplant recipients often need to limit high-phosphorus and high-potassium foods.

Caloric Requirements:

Meeting individual caloric needs ensures energy levels are sustained, supporting recovery and preventing malnutrition.

Monitoring and Individualization:

Regular Check-Ups:

Periodic assessments by healthcare professionals, including dietitians, are essential to monitor nutrient levels, kidney function, and overall health.

Tailoring the Diet:

Diet recommendations are not one-size-fits-all. Individual health conditions, medications, and personal preferences must be considered when crafting a post-transplant diet plan.

Emotional and Psychological Well-being:

Enjoying Food Safely:

A well-thought-out diet plan should not only address nutritional needs but also include enjoyable and flavorful options, promoting a positive relationship with food.

Mental Health Support:

The post-transplant period may bring about emotional challenges. Dietary adjustments should be accompanied by emotional support to ensure holistic well-being.

Chapter 1: Kidney Transplant Basics

Overview of Kidney Transplantation

Kidney transplantation is a transformative medical procedure that offers a new lease on life to individuals facing end-stage renal disease (ESRD) or other severe kidney conditions. This complex surgical intervention involves the replacement of a diseased or failed kidney with a healthy one from either a living or deceased donor. The process is marked by meticulous evaluation, surgical precision, and ongoing post-transplant care. Here's a comprehensive overview of the key facets of kidney transplantation:

1. Indications for Kidney Transplantation:

Kidney transplantation becomes a consideration when conventional treatments, such as medications and dialysis, are no longer effective in managing kidney dysfunction. Common indications include ESRD, irreversible kidney damage, or certain genetic disorders affecting the kidneys.

2. The Transplantation Process:

Donor Matching: Potential donors undergo thorough assessments to ensure compatibility with the recipient. Living donors, often family members or friends, undergo comprehensive evaluations. Deceased donors contribute kidneys through organ donation programs.

Recipient Evaluation: Recipients are meticulously evaluated for general health, medical history, and potential risks. Blood and tissue typing are conducted to enhance compatibility between the donor and recipient.

3. Types of Kidney Transplants:

Living Donor Transplant: Involves the transplantation of a kidney from a living donor, typically a family member, friend, or altruistic individual.

Deceased Donor Transplant: The kidney is obtained from a deceased donor, often through organ donation programs.

4. The Transplant Surgery:

The surgical procedure involves removing the damaged or failed kidney and replacing it with the healthy donor kidney. The surgeon connects the new kidney's blood vessels to the recipient's blood vessels and attaches the ureter to the bladder.

5. Immunosuppressive Medications:

Post-transplant, recipients are prescribed immunosuppressive medications to prevent rejection of the transplanted organ. These medications suppress the immune system's response to minimize the risk of the body attacking the new kidney.

6. Post-Transplant Recovery and Care:

After the surgery, recipients undergo a period of recovery, often in a hospital setting. Regular monitoring, including routine check-ups, is essential to ensure the transplanted kidney functions optimally. Medications are adjusted based on individual response and requirements.

7. Complications and Risks:

While kidney transplantation is generally successful, there are potential complications, including rejection, infections, and side effects of immunosuppressive medications. Ongoing medical follow-ups and adherence to prescribed medications help manage and mitigate these risks.

8. Long-Term Outcomes:

Successful kidney transplantation can significantly enhance the recipient's quality of life. Many recipients experience restored kidney function, reduced reliance on dialysis, and the opportunity to lead more active and fulfilling lives.

9. The Gift of Life:

Kidney transplantation represents a profound gift of life, showcasing the generosity of donors and the dedication of healthcare professionals committed to improving the well-being of individuals facing kidney-related challenges.

10. Advancements in Transplantation Research:

Ongoing research continues to explore ways to improve transplantation outcomes, reduce the need for immunosuppressive medications, and investigate alternative sources for donor organs.

In essence, kidney transplantation is a remarkable medical achievement that not only addresses the physical challenges of kidney disease but also brings hope, renewed vitality, and the promise of an improved quality of life for everyone undergoing this transformative procedure. As medical science advances, the landscape of kidney transplantation evolves, offering hope for a brighter future for individuals in need of this life-changing intervention.

Post-Transplant Dietary Guidelines

After undergoing a kidney transplant, adopting a thoughtful and kidney-friendly diet becomes crucial for the success of the transplant and the overall well-being of the recipient. The following dietary guidelines are designed to support a healthy and balanced lifestyle post-transplant:

1. Hydration:

Importance: Adequate hydration is essential for kidney function and overall health.

Guidelines: Consume an appropriate amount of fluids daily. However, consult with healthcare professionals to determine personalized fluid goals.

2. Sodium Control:

Importance: Managing sodium intake helps regulate blood pressure and prevent fluid retention.

Guidelines: Limit high-sodium foods, such as processed foods, canned soups, and salty snacks. Opt for fresh and whole foods, and use herbs and spices for flavoring.

3. Protein Intake:

Importance: Protein is crucial for healing but needs to be balanced to avoid overtaxing the kidneys.

Guidelines: Consume moderate amounts of high-quality protein sources such as lean meats, poultry, fish, eggs, and plant-based proteins. Consult with a dietitian to determine individual protein needs.

4. Phosphorus and Potassium Regulation:

Importance: Monitoring phosphorus and potassium levels helps prevent complications.

Guidelines: Limit high-phosphorus foods like dairy products and processed foods. Manage potassium intake by choosing low-potassium fruits and vegetables and avoiding salt substitutes containing potassium.

5. Calcium Intake:

Importance: Adequate calcium supports bone health, especially considering the potential impact of immunosuppressive medications.

Guidelines: Include calcium-rich foods like low-fat dairy, fortified plant-based milk, and leafy greens in the diet.

6. Limiting Oxalate-Rich Foods:

Importance: High oxalate levels can contribute to kidney stone formation.

Guidelines: Limit foods high in oxalates, such as beets, chocolate, nuts, and certain leafy greens. However, individual tolerance may vary.

7. Food Safety:

Importance: Post-transplant individuals are more susceptible to infections, necessitating attention to food safety.

Guidelines: Practice proper food handling, washing hands before meals, and avoiding raw or undercooked meats and unpasteurized dairy.

8. Vitamin and Mineral Supplements:

Importance: Some recipients may require supplements due to potential nutrient deficiencies.

Guidelines: Work with healthcare professionals to assess and address any specific nutritional needs through appropriate supplements.

9. Balanced Meals:

Importance: Well-balanced meals provide essential nutrients for overall health.

Guidelines: Include a variety of fruits, vegetables, whole grains, and lean proteins in each meal to ensure a diverse nutrient intake.

10. Regular Monitoring and Adjustments:

Importance: Individual nutritional needs may change over time, requiring periodic adjustments.

Guidelines: Regularly consult with a registered dietitian or healthcare team to assess dietary requirements, making necessary modifications based on health status and medications.

11. Weight Management:

Importance: Maintaining a healthy weight supports overall health and may help manage potential side effects of immunosuppressive medications.

Guidelines: Work with healthcare professionals to establish and maintain a healthy weight through a combination of a balanced diet and regular physical activity.

Chapter 2: Breakfast Delights

1. Spinach and Feta Omelette:

Ingredients:

- Eggs

- Fresh spinach

- Feta cheese (low in sodium)

- Olive oil

- Salt and pepper to taste

Instructions:

- Whisk eggs in a bowl and season with salt and pepper.

- Sauté fresh spinach in your olive oil until wilted.

- Pour whisked eggs over spinach in a pan.

- Sprinkle crumbled feta on top.

- Cook until the eggs are set, then fold and serve.

2. Blueberry Almond Smoothie Bowl:

Ingredients:

- Frozen blueberries

- Almond milk

- Greek yogurt

- Almond butter

- Honey

Instructions:

- Blend frozen blueberries, almond milk, Greek yogurt, and almond butter until smooth.

- Pour into a bowl and drizzle with honey.

- Top with sliced almonds for added crunch.

3. Chia Seed Pudding with Berries:

Ingredients:

- Chia seeds

- Almond milk

- Mixed berries (strawberries, blueberries, raspberries)

- Vanilla extract

- Maple syrup

Instructions:

- Mix chia seeds with almond milk, vanilla extract, and a touch of maple syrup.

- Refrigerate overnight.

- Top with fresh mixed berries before serving.

4. Banana Nut Quinoa Bowl:

Ingredients:

- Cooked quinoa

- Sliced bananas

- Chopped walnuts

- Cinnamon

- Honey

Instructions:

- Combine cooked quinoa, sliced bananas, and chopped walnuts in a bowl.

- Sprinkle with cinnamon and drizzle with honey.

5. Greek Yogurt Parfait with Granola:

Ingredients:

- Greek yogurt

- Mixed berries

- Low-phosphorus granola

- Honey

Instructions:

• Layer Greek yogurt with mixed berries in a glass.

• Top with a sprinkle of low-phosphorus granola. Drizzle with honey.

6. Oatmeal with Sliced Almonds and Berries:

Ingredients:

• Rolled oats

• Almond milk

• Sliced almonds

• Mixed berries

• Cinnamon

Instructions:

- Cook rolled oats in almond milk.

- Top with sliced almonds, mixed berries, and a dash of cinnamon.

7. Low-Phosphorus Pancakes:

Ingredients:

- Whole wheat flour

- Baking powder

- Almond milk

- Egg whites

- Vanilla extract

Instructions:

- Mix whole wheat flour, baking powder, almond milk, egg whites, and vanilla extract to make a pancake batter.

- Cook on a griddle until golden brown.

8. Breakfast Quinoa Bowl with Apples and Cinnamon:

Ingredients:

- Cooked quinoa

- Sliced apples

- Chopped pecans

- Cinnamon and Maple syrup

Instructions:

- Combine cooked quinoa, sliced apples, and chopped pecans in a bowl.

- Sprinkle it with cinnamon and drizzle it with maple syrup.

9. Buckwheat Pancakes with Berries:

Ingredients:

- Buckwheat flour

- Almond milk

- Egg whites

- Mixed berries

- Agave syrup

Instructions:

• Mix buckwheat flour, almond milk, and egg whites to make pancake batter.

• Cook on a griddle and top with mixed berries. Drizzle with agave syrup.

10. Smoothie Bowl with Mango and Coconut:

Ingredients:

• Frozen mango chunks

• Coconut milk

• Greek yogurt

• Chia seeds

• Shredded coconut

Instructions:

- Blend frozen mango, coconut milk, and Greek yogurt until smooth.

- Pour into a bowl and sprinkle with chia seeds and shredded coconut.

Always consult with healthcare professionals or a dietitian to ensure that these breakfast options align with individual dietary needs and restrictions. Adjustments can be made based on personal health requirements.

Chapter 3: Lunchtime Favorites

1. Grilled Lemon Herb Chicken Salad:

Ingredients:

- Chicken breast

- Mixed salad greens

- Cherry tomatoes

- Cucumber

- Lemon

- Olive oil

- Fresh herbs (rosemary, thyme, or parsley)

Instructions:

● Season chicken breast with fresh herbs, lemon juice, and a drizzle of olive oil.

● Grill until fully cooked.

● Slice the grilled chicken and serve over a bed of mixed salad greens, cherry tomatoes, and sliced cucumber.

2. Quinoa and Vegetable Stuffed Bell Peppers:

Ingredients:

● Quinoa

● Bell peppers

● Zucchini

- Cherry tomatoes

- Red onion

- Feta cheese (optional)

Instructions:

- Cook quinoa according to package instructions.

- Mix cooked quinoa with diced zucchini, cherry tomatoes, red onion, and feta cheese.

- Stuff halved bell peppers with the quinoa mixture and bake until peppers are tender.

3. Tuna and White Bean Wrap:

Ingredients:

- Canned tuna (in water)

- White beans

- Whole wheat tortilla

- Spinach

- Red onion

- Greek yogurt

Instructions:

- Drain canned tuna and mix with white beans, diced red onion, and Greek yogurt.

- Spoon the tuna mixture onto a whole wheat tortilla, add spinach, and wrap.

4. Vegetable Stir-Fry with Tofu:

Ingredients:

- Tofu

- Broccoli

- Bell peppers

- Snap peas

- Carrots

- Low-sodium soy sauce

Instructions:

● Press and cube tofu, then stir-fry until golden.

● Add broccoli, bell peppers, snap peas, and carrots to the pan.

● Drizzle with low-sodium soy sauce and stir until vegetables are tender.

5. Lemon Herb Tilapia with Quinoa:

Ingredients:

● Tilapia fillets

● Quinoa

● Lemon

- Fresh herbs (parsley, dill)

- Olive oil

Instructions:

- Season tilapia fillets with fresh herbs, lemon juice, and olive oil.

- Bake or grill it until the fish is cooked through.

- Serve over a bed of cooked quinoa.

6. Turkey and Vegetable Skewers:

Ingredients:

- Ground turkey

- Zucchini

- Cherry tomatoes

- Red onion

- Olive oil

- Garlic powder

Instructions:

- Mix ground turkey with garlic powder and form into skewers.

• Alternate threading skewers with zucchini, cherry tomatoes, and red onion.

• Grill until turkey is cooked through and vegetables are tender.

7. Mediterranean Chickpea Salad:

Ingredients:

• Chickpeas

• Cucumber

• Cherry tomatoes

• Kalamata olives

• Feta cheese (optional)

• Olive oil and Lemon juice

Instructions:

- Combine chickpeas, diced cucumber, cherry tomatoes, Kalamata olives, and feta cheese.

- Drizzle with olive oil and lemon juice. Toss until well combined.

8. Spinach and Strawberry Salad with Balsamic Vinaigrette:

Ingredients:

- Fresh spinach

- Strawberries

- Goat cheese (optional)

- Walnuts

- Balsamic vinaigrette dressing

Instructions:

- Toss fresh spinach with sliced strawberries, crumbled goat cheese, and walnuts.

- Drizzle with balsamic vinaigrette dressing.

9. Brown Rice and Black Bean Bowl:

Ingredients:

- Brown rice

- Black beans

- Corn

- Avocado

- Salsa

Instructions:

- Cook brown rice according to package instructions.

- Mix cooked rice with black beans, corn, diced avocado, and salsa.

10. Roasted Eggplant and Tomato Pasta:

Ingredients:

- Whole wheat pasta

- Eggplant

- Cherry tomatoes

- Garlic

- Olive oil

- Fresh basil

Instructions:

- Roast eggplant, cherry tomatoes, and garlic with olive oil in the oven.

- Toss roasted vegetables with cooked whole wheat pasta.

- Garnish with fresh basil before serving.

Chapter 4: Satisfying Snacks

1. Cucumber and Hummus Bites:

Ingredients:

- Cucumber

- Hummus

- Cherry tomatoes (optional)

Instructions:

- Slice cucumber into rounds.

- Top each cucumber round with a small dollop of hummus.

• Garnish with a halved cherry tomato if desired.

2. Baked Apple Chips:

Ingredients:

• Apples

• Cinnamon

• Nutmeg (optional)

Instructions:

• Slice apples thinly.

• Arrange slices on a baking sheet and sprinkle with cinnamon (and nutmeg if desired).

- Bake it at a low temperature until crisp.

3. Rice Cake with Almond Butter and Banana Slices:

Ingredients:

- Rice cake

- Almond butter

- Banana

Instructions:

- Spread almond butter on a rice cake.

- Top with banana slices.

4. Greek Yogurt with Berries and Granola:

Ingredients:

- Greek yogurt

- Mixed berries

- Low-phosphorus granola

Instructions:

- Spoon Greek yogurt into a bowl.

- Top with mixed berries and a sprinkle of low-phosphorus granola.

5. Trail Mix with Nuts and Seeds (in moderation):

Ingredients:

- Almonds

- Walnuts

- Pumpkin seeds

- Dried cranberries (unsweetened)

Instructions:

- Combine almonds, walnuts, pumpkin seeds, and dried cranberries in a bowl.

- Mix well and portion into small servings.

6. Celery Sticks with Peanut Butter:

Ingredients:

- Celery sticks

- Peanut butter (unsalted)

Instructions:

- Spread peanut butter onto celery sticks.

7. Baked Sweet Potato Fries:

Ingredients:

- Sweet potatoes

- Olive oil

- Paprika

Instructions:

- Cut sweet potatoes into fry shapes.

- Toss with olive oil and paprika.

- Bake until crispy.

8. Cherry Tomato Bruschetta:

Ingredients:

- Cherry tomatoes

- Whole-grain crackers

- Basil

- Balsamic glaze

Instructions:

- Slice cherry tomatoes and place them on whole-grain crackers.

- Garnish with fresh basil and drizzle with balsamic glaze.

9. Cottage Cheese and Pineapple Cups:

Ingredients:

- Low-fat cottage cheese

- Pineapple chunks

Instructions:

- Scoop low-fat cottage cheese into small cups.

- Top with pineapple chunks.

10. Edamame with Sea Salt:

Ingredients:

- Edamame (steamed)

- Sea salt

Instructions:

- Steam edamame according to package instructions.

- Sprinkle with sea salt before serving.

Chapter 5: Dinner Delicacies

1. Grilled Lemon Herb Chicken:

Ingredients:

- Chicken breasts

- Lemon

- Fresh herbs (rosemary, thyme)

- Olive oil

- Garlic

Instructions:

• Marinate chicken breasts in a mixture of lemon juice, fresh herbs, minced garlic, and olive oil.

• Grill until fully cooked.

2. Quinoa and Vegetable Stir-Fry:

Ingredients:

• Quinoa

• Mixed vegetables (broccoli, bell peppers, carrots)

• Low-sodium soy sauce

• Ginger and Garlic

Instructions:

• Cook quinoa according to package instructions.

• Stir-fry mixed vegetables with ginger and garlic.

• Toss cooked quinoa into the stir-fried vegetables and add low-sodium soy sauce.

3. Lemon Herb Tilapia with Brown Rice:

Ingredients:

• Tilapia fillets

• Lemon

• Fresh herbs (dill, parsley)

* Olive oil

* Brown rice

Instructions:

* Season tilapia fillets with fresh herbs, lemon juice, and olive oil.

* Bake or grill it until the fish is cooked through.

* Serve over a bed of cooked brown rice.

4. Mediterranean Chickpea and Spinach Stew:

Ingredients:

- Chickpeas

- Spinach

- Tomatoes

- Garlic

- Olive oil

- Cumin

Instructions:

- Sauté garlic in your olive oil until fragrant.

- Add chickpeas, chopped tomatoes, and cumin.

- Simmer until the stew thickens, then stir in fresh spinach.

5. Turkey and Vegetable Skewers with Quinoa:

Ingredients:

- Ground turkey

- Zucchini

- Cherry tomatoes

- Quinoa

- Olive oil

- Italian seasoning

Instructions:

- Mix ground turkey with Italian seasoning and form into skewers.

- Alternate threading skewers with zucchini and cherry tomatoes.

- Grill until turkey is cooked through.

- Serve over a bed of cooked quinoa.

6. Roasted Eggplant and Tomato Pasta:

Ingredients:

- Whole wheat pasta

- Eggplant

- Cherry tomatoes

- Garlic

- Olive oil

- Fresh basil

Instructions:

- Roast eggplant, cherry tomatoes, and garlic with olive oil in the oven.

- Toss roasted vegetables with cooked whole wheat pasta.

- Garnish with fresh basil before serving.

7. Mashed Cauliflower with Grilled Chicken:

Ingredients:

- Cauliflower

- Chicken breast

- Olive oil

- Garlic

- Low-sodium chicken broth

Instructions:

- Steam cauliflower until tender.

- Mash cauliflower with minced garlic and a splash of low-sodium chicken broth.

• Grill chicken breast and serve over the mashed cauliflower.

8. Sautéed Green Beans with Lemon:

Ingredients:

• Fresh green beans

• Lemon

• Olive oil

• Garlic

Instructions:

• Sauté green beans in olive oil until crisp-tender.

• Add minced garlic and then cook until fragrant.

• Squeeze lemon juice over the green beans before serving.

9. Quinoa Pilaf with Mixed Vegetables:

Ingredients:

• Quinoa

• Mixed vegetables (bell peppers, peas, carrots)

• Onion

• Olive oil

Instructions:

- Cook quinoa according to package instructions.

- Sauté mixed vegetables and onion in olive oil.

- Mix cooked quinoa with sautéed vegetables to create a pilaf.

10. Roasted Brussels Sprouts with Baked Salmon:

Ingredients:

- Brussels sprouts

- Salmon fillets

- Olive oil

- Lemon

- Garlic

Instructions:

• Toss Brussels sprouts with olive oil and roast until crispy.

• Season salmon fillets with minced garlic and lemon juice, then bake until cooked through.

Chapter 6: Side Dishes to Savor

1. Mashed Cauliflower:

Ingredients:

- Cauliflower

- Olive oil

- Garlic

- Low-sodium chicken broth

Instructions:

- Steam cauliflower until tender.

- Mash cauliflower with minced garlic and a splash of low-sodium chicken broth.

2. Sautéed Green Beans:

Ingredients:

● Fresh green beans

● Olive oil

● Garlic

Instructions:

● Sauté green beans in olive oil until crisp-tender.

● Add minced garlic and then cook until fragrant.

3. Quinoa Pilaf with Mixed Vegetables:

Ingredients:

• Quinoa

• Mixed vegetables (bell peppers, peas, carrots)

• Onion

• Olive oil

Instructions:

• Cook quinoa according to package instructions.

• Sauté mixed vegetables and onion in olive oil.

- Mix cooked quinoa with sautéed vegetables to create a pilaf.

4. Roasted Brussels Sprouts:

Ingredients:

- Brussels sprouts

- Olive oil

- Garlic

Instructions:

- Toss Brussels sprouts with olive oil and roast until crispy.

- Add minced garlic for added flavor.

5. Sautéed Spinach with Lemon:

Ingredients:

- Fresh spinach

- Olive oil

- Lemon

- Garlic

Instructions:

- Sauté fresh spinach in your olive oil until wilted.

- Add minced garlic and squeeze lemon juice over the spinach.

6. Baked Sweet Potato Fries:

Ingredients:

- Sweet potatoes

- Olive oil

- Paprika

Instructions:

- Cut sweet potatoes into fry shapes.

- Toss with olive oil and paprika.

- Bake until crispy.

7. Cucumber and Tomato Salad:

Ingredients:

- Cucumber

- Cherry tomatoes

- Red onion

- Olive oil

- Balsamic vinegar

- Fresh basil

Instructions:

- Dice cucumber, cherry tomatoes, and red onion.

- Toss with olive oil, balsamic vinegar, and fresh basil.

8. Quinoa and Black Bean Salad:

Ingredients:

- Quinoa

- Black beans

- Corn

- Bell peppers

- Cilantro

- Lime

Instructions:

- Cook quinoa according to package instructions.

- Mix cooked quinoa with black beans, corn, diced bell peppers, chopped cilantro, and lime juice.

9. Steamed Asparagus with Lemon:

Ingredients:

- Fresh asparagus

- Lemon

- Olive oil

Instructions:

● Steam asparagus until tender.

● Drizzle with olive oil and squeeze lemon juice over the top.

10. Cauliflower Rice:

Ingredients:

● Cauliflower

● Olive oil

● Garlic

● Salt and pepper

Instructions:

- Grate or process cauliflower in to rice-sized pieces.

- Sauté in olive oil with your minced garlic until tender.

- Season with salt and pepper to taste.

Chapter 7: Desserts for Joy

1. Baked Apples with Cinnamon:

Ingredients:

- Apples

- Cinnamon

- Nutmeg (optional)

Instructions:

- Core apples and sprinkle with cinnamon (and nutmeg if desired).

- Bake until tender.

2. Berry Sorbet:

Ingredients:

- Mixed berries (strawberries, blueberries, raspberries)

- Honey

- Lemon juice

Instructions:

- Blend mixed berries, honey, and lemon juice until smooth.

- Freeze the mixture in an ice cream maker or a shallow dish, stirring occasionally.

3. Angel Food Cake with Fresh Fruit:

Ingredients:

- Angel food cake

- Mixed fresh fruit (berries, kiwi, pineapple)

- Whipped cream (optional)

Instructions:

- Slice angel food cake and top with mixed fresh fruit.

- Garnish with a dollop of whipped cream if desired.

4. Pumpkin Pudding:

Ingredients:

- Canned pumpkin

- Greek yogurt

- Pumpkin spice

- Maple syrup

Instructions:

- Mix canned pumpkin with Greek yogurt, pumpkin spice, and maple syrup.

- Chill in the refrigerator before serving.

5. Coconut Rice Pudding:

Ingredients:

- Arborio rice

- Coconut milk

- Coconut flakes

- Vanilla extract

- Maple syrup

Instructions:

- Cook Arborio rice in coconut milk until creamy.

- Stir in coconut flakes, vanilla extract, and maple syrup.

6. Low-Phosphorus Pancakes with Berries:

Ingredients:

- Whole wheat flour

- Baking powder

- Almond milk

- Egg whites

- Vanilla extract

- Mixed berries

Instructions:

- Mix whole wheat flour, baking powder, almond milk, egg whites, and vanilla extract to make a pancake batter.

- Cook on a griddle until golden brown.

- Top with mixed berries.

7. Herbal Iced Tea:

Ingredients:

- Herbal tea bags

- Water

- Lemon

- Fresh mint

- Honey (optional)

Instructions:

- Brew your herbal tea and let it cool.

- Add lemon slices, fresh mint, and sweeten with honey if desired.

- Serve over ice.

8. Cranberry Spritzer:

Ingredients:

- Cranberry juice (unsweetened)

- Sparkling water

- Lime

- Ice

Instructions:

- Mix unsweetened cranberry juice with sparkling water.

• Add a squeeze of lime and serve over ice.

9. Watermelon Mint Cooler:

Ingredients:

• Fresh watermelon

• Fresh mint

• Lime

• Ice

Instructions:

• Blend fresh watermelon until smooth.

• Add chopped mint, a squeeze of lime, and serve over ice.

10. Cherry Almond Smoothie:

Ingredients:

- Frozen cherries

- Almond milk

- Greek yogurt

- Almond extract

- Honey

Instructions:

- Blend frozen cherries, almond milk, Greek yogurt, almond extract, and honey until smooth.

Chapter 8: Beverages for Refreshment

1. Herbal Iced Tea:

Ingredients:

- Herbal tea bags (caffeine-free)

- Water

- Lemon slices

- Fresh mint

- Honey (optional)

Instructions:

- Brew your herbal tea and let it cool.

- Add lemon slices, fresh mint, and sweeten with honey if desired.

* Serve over ice.

2. Cranberry Spritzer:

Ingredients:

* Unsweetened cranberry juice

* Sparkling water

* Lime slices

* Ice

Instructions:

* Mix unsweetened cranberry juice with sparkling water.

* Add lime slices and serve over ice.

3. Watermelon Mint Cooler:

Ingredients:

- Fresh watermelon

- Fresh mint leaves

- Lime juice

- Ice

Instructions:

- Blend fresh watermelon until smooth.

- Add chopped mint leaves and a squeeze of lime.

- Serve over ice.

4. Ginger Lemonade:

Ingredients:

- Fresh ginger

- Lemon juice

- Water

- Honey (optional)

- Ice

Instructions:

- Grate fresh ginger and mix with lemon juice.

- Dilute with water, sweeten with honey if desired, and serve over ice.

5. Cherry Almond Smoothie:

Ingredients:

- Frozen cherries

- Almond milk

- Greek yogurt

- Almond extract

- Honey

Instructions:

- Blend frozen cherries, almond milk, Greek yogurt, almond extract, and honey until smooth.

6. Low-Phosphorus Fruit Punch:

Ingredients:

- Pineapple juice (unsweetened)

- Orange juice (unsweetened)

- Apple juice (unsweetened)

- Sparkling water

- Ice

Instructions:

- Mix equal parts pineapple juice, orange juice, and apple juice.

- Dilute with sparkling water and serve over ice.

7. Coconut Water with Lime:

Ingredients:

- Coconut water

- Lime slices

- Ice

Instructions:

- Pour coconut water over ice.

- Add lime slices for a refreshing twist.

8. Minty Cucumber Cooler:

Ingredients:

- Cucumber slices

- Fresh mint leaves

- Lime juice

- Sparkling water

- Ice

Instructions:

- Muddle cucumber slices and mint leaves.

- Add your lime juice, sparkling water, and ice.

9. Cherry Berry Iced Tea:

Ingredients:

• Mixed berry herbal tea bags

• Water

• Frozen mixed berries

• Lemon slices

• Ice

Instructions:

• Brew mixed berry herbal tea and let it cool.

• Add frozen mixed berries, lemon slices, and serve over ice.

10. Pineapple Mint Sparkler:

Ingredients:

- Pineapple juice (unsweetened)

- Fresh mint leaves

- Sparkling water

- Ice

Instructions:

- Mix pineapple juice with fresh mint leaves.

- Dilute with sparkling water and serve over ice.

Conclusion

"The Complete Kidney Transplant Diet Cookbook" aims to be an invaluable resource for individuals navigating the intricate path of post-kidney transplant dietary guidelines. This comprehensive guide has endeavored to provide a diverse array of recipes and meal plans tailored to meet the unique nutritional needs of transplant patients.

Our journey through this cookbook has explored flavorsome breakfast delights, satisfying lunchtime favorites, delectable dinner delicacies, tantalizing side dishes, and joyful desserts, all meticulously crafted to align with the dietary considerations crucial for kidney transplant recipients. Additionally, we've ventured into refreshing beverages and invigorating snacks, offering a holistic approach to maintaining a balanced and enjoyable diet.

Throughout these pages, a commitment to kidney-friendly ingredients, mindful cooking methods, and delicious results is evident. The recipes are not just about nourishment; they are a celebration of the joy that food can bring, even within the constraints of a post-transplant diet.

As you embark on your culinary journey with "The Complete Kidney Transplant Diet Cookbook," remember that each recipe is a testament to the fusion of health and taste. However, it's imperative to consult with healthcare professionals or a dietitian to ensure that these recipes align with your individual health requirements. Here's to savoring every bite on the road to wellness and embracing the transformative power of a nourishing, delightful diet after kidney transplantation.